CURING BIPOLAR DISORDER

AND SCHIZOPHRENIA

CURING BIPOLAR DISORDER AND SCHIZOPHRENIA

A STEP-BY-STEP GUIDE TO RECOVERY AND WELLNESS

DORIS KING, CMHP

EVE PUBLISHING

FLORIDA

This book is not intended to replace a one-on-one relationship with a qualified healthcare professional. This book should be used as an informational guide only and should not be considered as medical advice. The information contained in this book is based on the research and experience of the author. You should consult your medical professional regarding issues pertaining to your health, especially relating to the diagnosis of a disease or to any symptoms that you may be experiencing.

Copyright © 2009 by Doris King, CMHP. All rights reserved. Except as permitted under the U.S. Copyright Act of 1976, no part of this publication may be reproduced, distributed, or transmitted in any form or by any means, or stored in a database or retrieval system, without the written permission of the publisher.

Eve Publishing
P.O. Box 289
Lake Alfred, Florida 33850

Visit our Web site at www.evepublishing.com

First Edition: September 2009

Designed by Rodrigo Corral

Printed on acid-free paper in the United States of America and the United Kingdom

Library of Congress Control Number: 2009934964

ISBN: 978-0-982-4853-0-9

10 9 8 7 6 5 4 3 2 1

This book is dedicated to everyone who has bipolar disorder and schizophrenia, and their families

Contents

CHAPTER 1
Introduction 10

CHAPTER 2
Understanding Your Symptoms 12

CHAPTER 3
What is Progesterone? 16

CHAPTER 4
Curing Bipolar Disorder and Schizophrenia 23

CHAPTER 5
Recovery Step-by-Step 40

CHAPTER 6
Finding a Doctor 57

CHAPTER 7
Questions and Answers 61

CONCLUSION 73

RESOURCES 74

REFERENCES 80

INDEX 94

ABOUT THE AUTHOR 101

1
INTRODUCTION

The National Institute of Mental Health estimates that 8 million Americans suffer from bipolar disorder or schizophrenia. I used to be one of them.

I'm not going to go into much detail about my illness, but I will tell you that I suffered from symptoms of both disorders. And like most people with mental illness, I thought I would die with my disease.

But I don't have that grim outlook anymore. Today I live symptom-free.

My outlook on life changed in 2006. That fall, I discovered the work of the late Dr. John Lee. Dr. Lee was a brilliant family doctor who wrote several books on hormone balance.

In his book, *Hormone Balance Made Simple*, Dr. Lee listed a group of symptoms that were caused by low progesterone levels. I read through his list and realized I had most of the symptoms.

Headaches: check. Fibrocystic breasts: check. Fatigue: check. Irritability: check, check, check!

It was clear my body needed progesterone.

I followed Dr. Lee's advice and corrected my progesterone deficiency. At the time, I had no idea I was going to "recover" from mental illness. I was taking progesterone to get rid of my headaches and fatigue.

Those symptoms went away —as did my symptoms of mental illness. My thoughts slowed down, the voices I heard stopped, my emotions became stable, and I slept through the night for the first time in years.

All of these wonderful things were happening in my body because of progesterone.

Since discovering its benefits, I've been dedicated to telling others about it.

In this book, I will help you determine if low progesterone levels are making you sick. Then I will give you the resources you'll need to correct it.

Let's begin.

2
UNDERSTANDING YOUR SYMPTOMS

Before we get into why your body needs progesterone, we will need to go over common symptoms of bipolar disorder and schizophrenia. Then, we can trace each symptom back to progesterone.

Bipolar Symptoms

When you have bipolar disorder, you live between extremes — mania and depression.

Mania is the "up" phase of bipolar disorder. When you are manic you may not realize you're sick. Many people become more productive when they're manic, accomplishing most things they set out to do.

Depression is the "down" phase of bipolar disorder. When you are depressed, you feel the opposite of when you are manic. During depression, it's common to have low energy and you may have difficulty completing simple tasks.

Other symptoms common to mania and depression are listed below:

MANIA SYMPTOMS INCLUDE:

- Extremely high energy levels
- Racing thoughts
- Feeling pressure to talk
- Talking too much or too loud
- A decreased need for sleep
- Elevated mood
- Increased activity level
- Inflated self-esteem
- Unrealistic beliefs in your abilities
- Poor impulse control (this can lead to overspending, sexual indiscretions, poor business decisions, and substance abuse)
- Irritability

DEPRESSION SYMPTOMS INCLUDE:

- A sad, empty mood
- Uncontrollable crying
- Changes in appetite and weight
- A fatigue that doesn't improve with sleep
- Losing interest in things you once enjoyed
- Poor concentration
- Difficulty recalling information or making decisions
- Sleeping too much
- Feelings of guilt or worthlessness
- Believing you are a burden to your friends and family
- Thoughts of death or suicide or making plans to die

Symptoms of mania and depression can wreak havoc on your life, because you don't always know how you're going to feel one moment to the next. This can cause problems for you at work or school and in your relationships.

Schizophrenia

When you have schizophrenia, it's common to experience symptoms of mania and depression, and problems with your thoughts and senses as well.

- When your thoughts are altered, this is known as **delusion**.
- When your senses are altered, this is called **hallucination**.
- A delusion is when you believe something is true when it's not.
- When you hallucinate, you hear, see, smell, taste, or feel things that no one else can.

Common delusions and hallucinations are listed below:

COMMON DELUSIONS INCLUDE:

- Believing you have special powers or knowledge that no one else has
- Thinking you are psychic or have mystical abilities
- Believing messages are being sent to you through the television or radio
- Thinking someone is out to get you or your family and do you harm

COMMON HALLUCINATIONS INCLUDE:

- Hearing voices. You may hear your own voice or the voices of others
- Seeing people. They may be dead or alive
- Tasting things differently as if they've been poisoned
- Smelling sweet, sickly odors
- Feeling things crawling on your skin

UNDERSTANDING YOUR SYMPTOMS 15

DELUSIONS AND HALLUCINATIONS ARE NOT THE ONLY SYMPTOMS OF SCHIZOPHRENIA. OTHER SYMPTOMS INCLUDE:

- Difficulty expressing your thoughts or feelings
- Loss of interest in activities you normally enjoy
- Memory problems
- Difficulty understanding people
- Uncontrollable rage or anger
- Difficulty caring for yourself
  (i.e., washing your hair, brushing your teeth)
- Social isolation
- Loss of motivation
- Problems making sense of information
- Clumsy uncoordinated movements
- Fatigue

Schizophrenia is usually the more debilitating of the two disorders. It can interfere with your ability to be gainfully employed. The most severe cases can require long-term hospitalization.

Symptoms of mental illness are caused by the body not having sufficient progesterone.

3
WHAT IS PROGESTERONE?

Progesterone is a hormone that helps you to maintain a healthy mind. For a long time, it was believed to be a female-only hormone, but it's not. Progesterone is made by both men and women for their mental health.

In this chapter we will focus on progesterone's role in the brain and adrenal glands. And then we will take a look at what happens when the brain and adrenals don't have the progesterone they need.

Progesterone and the Brain

Your brain controls every experience you can have in life. It helps you read, cough, run, laugh, and show affection.

A network of cells called *nerve cells* or *neurons* controls all your brain functions. Nerve cells do this by exchanging chemical and electrical signals. Progesterone helps your brain exchange these signals clearly. Below is an image of your brain.

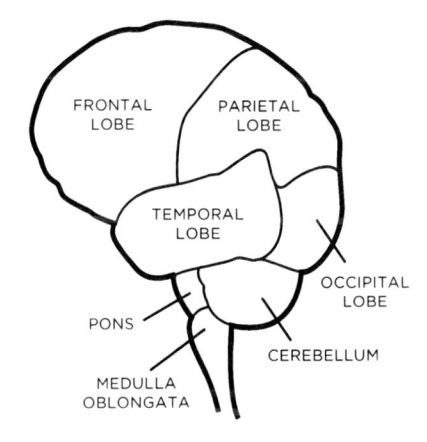

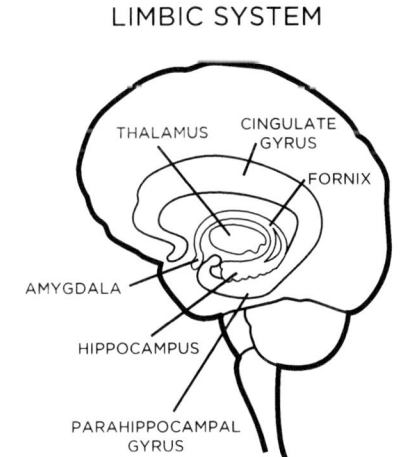

As you can see, your brain is made of many parts; each section controls a different aspect of your behavior.

YOUR FRONTAL LOBE CONTROLS:
- Planning
- Decision making
- Impulse control
- Reasoning

YOUR PARIETAL LOBE CONTROLS:
- Memory

YOUR TEMPORAL LOBES CONTROL:
- Hearing

YOUR OCCIPITAL LOBE CONTROLS:
- Vision

YOUR CEREBELLUM CONTROLS:
- Walking
- Talking
- Eating
- Balance and posture
- Grooming (showering, brushing your teeth)

YOUR BRAIN STEM (PONS, MEDULLA OBLONGATA) CONTROLS AUTONOMIC FUNCTIONS SUCH AS:
- Breathing
- Sneezing
- Coughing
- Blood pressure

The limbic system is responsible for processing your emotions. It's sometimes called the "emotional brain."

THE LIMBIC SYSTEM HELPS YOU EXPERIENCE FEELINGS OF:
- Happiness
- Sadness
- Anger
- Excitement
- Fear

IT ALSO CONTROLS:
- Humor
- Motivation
- Appetite
- Your ability to smell
- Your response to stress
- Social interactions

Progesterone helps your brain control its functions.

The Bipolar and Schizophrenic Brain

When you have bipolar disorder or schizophrenia, your brain doesn't have the progesterone it needs to function properly. This causes you to develop symptoms.

The symptoms that you experience will depend on the part of your brain that is having problems communicating. Let's take a look at some of these symptoms.

BROKEN COMMUNICATION IN THE FRONTAL LOBE CAUSES:
- Scattered thinking
- Personality changes
- Poor impulse control

BROKEN COMMUNICATION IN THE PARIETAL LOBE CAUSES:
- Memory problems

BROKEN COMMUNICATION IN THE TEMPORAL LOBES CAUSE:
- Hallucinations of sound (auditory hallucinations)

BROKEN COMMUNICATION IN THE OCCIPITAL LOBE CAUSES:
- Hallucinations of sight (visual hallucinations)

BROKEN COMMUNICATION IN THE CEREBELLUM CAUSES:
- Difficulty grooming
- Speech problems
- Involuntary movements

BROKEN COMMUNICATION IN THE BRAIN STEM CAN CAUSE:
- Confusion
- Behavior changes

WHEN YOUR LIMBIC SYSTEM CAN'T PROCESS INFORMATION CLEARLY, THIS CAUSES:
- Depression
- Inappropriate humor
- Irritability
- Anxiety disorders
- Unstable emotions
- Smelling things differently
- Paranoia
- Uncontrollable anger
- Problems interacting with others
- Changes in appetite
- Low motivation

Progesterone is the fuel of the brain. Just as a car can't run without gasoline, your brain can't run without progesterone.

Progesterone and the Adrenal Glands

Low levels of progesterone impact more than your brain. Your adrenal glands are also affected.

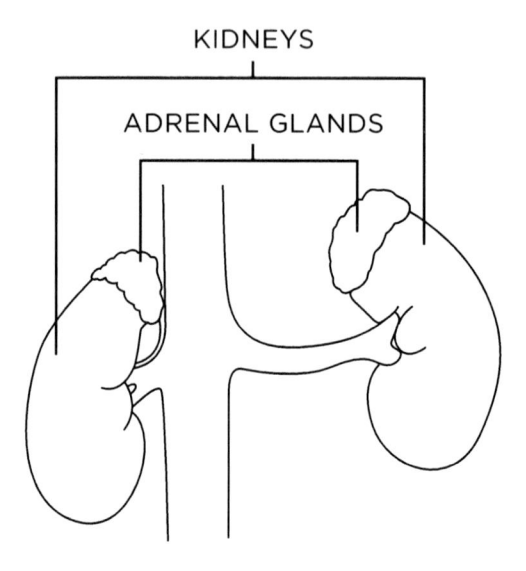

The adrenal glands are two triangular glands that sit on top of your kidneys. Your adrenal glands use progesterone to make the hormones cortisol and aldosterone. Cortisol and aldosterone control most adrenal gland processes.

WHAT IS PROGESTERONE? 21

CORTISOL AND ALDOSTERONE CONTROL:
- Energy levels (blood sugar)
- Concentration
- Your immune response
- Blood pressure
- Arousal
- Digestion
- Stress
- The release of adrenaline (epinephrine)

When you have mental illness, your cortisol and aldosterone levels are unbalanced because of low progesterone. This causes a syndrome known as *Adrenal Fatigue*.

SYMPTOMS OF ADRENAL FATIGUE INCLUDE:
- A fatigue that doesn't improve with sleep
- Difficulty waking in the morning
- Depression
- Irritability
- Poor concentration
- An overactive immune system (which can lead to autoimmune disease or swollen lymph nodes, i.e. adenoids and tonsils)
- Lightheadedness
- Low blood pressure
- Craving of sweet or salty foods
- Seizures, movement problems
- Heart palpitations
- Sleep disturbances (sleeping too much or too little)
- Anxiety disorders
- Mania (uncontrolled adrenaline release)

If you would like to know more about the physiology behind these disorders, you should read Dr. James Wilson's book *Adrenal Fatigue: The 21st Century Stress Syndrome* (Smart Publications, 2002).

Why isn't my body making enough progesterone?

Dr. Michael Glaser, Professor Emeritus of Biochemistry and Neuroscience at the University of Illinois, says the sex organs are responsible for making the bulk of the progesterone the brain uses.

So if your brain is not getting the progesterone it needs, that means your sex organs are not making enough of it. Female sex organs are called ovaries. Male sex organs are called testes.

When your sex organs aren't making sufficient amounts of a particular hormone, this is a medical condition known as *hypogonadism*.

Hypogonadism can refer to deficiencies in testosterone and estrogen as well. However, in the case of mental illness the deficiency pertains to progesterone.

When your sex organs can't make enough of the progesterone your brain needs, your brain begins to use the progesterone made by your adrenal glands.

Your adrenal glands make far less progesterone than your sex organs. Thus the adrenal glands are unable to meet the brain's demands. They burn out. Mental illness sets in.

Your body was never designed to function this way. It was designed to create sufficient progesterone so your brain and adrenal glands can work properly.

In order to correct what is happening in your body and restore your mental and physical health, you will need to give your body the progesterone it needs.

4

CURING BIPOLAR DISORDER AND SCHIZOPHRENIA

Giving your body a hormone it should have been producing is not as unusual as it seems. Type 1 or juvenile diabetes is a disease caused by the body not making enough insulin. That's why diabetics have to take insulin in order to prevent illness.

And the same must be done with progesterone. To learn how to take progesterone, you will need to follow the advice of Dr. Lee, just like I did.

This chapter is based on his work and research.

Dr. Lee's 3 Rules of Hormone Balance:

RULE 1: Take Progesterone Only if You Need It (e.g., if your levels are measurably low or if you have clear symptoms)
RULE 2: Take Bioidentical Progesterone Instead of Synthetic Progestins
RULE 3: Take Progesterone in Physiological Amounts Only

Reprinted by permission from The Official Web Site of Dr. John R. Lee, M.D. (www.JohnLeeMD.com)

Dr. Lee's rules are really easy to follow. If you stick to his rules, you will be on the right road to hormone balance. Let's go through each rule one by one.

RULE 1: TAKE PROGESTERONE ONLY IF YOU NEED IT (E.G., IF YOUR LEVELS ARE MEASURABLY LOW OR IF YOU HAVE CLEAR SYMPTOMS)

The good news is you don't have to guess whether or not your body is making enough progesterone. Progesterone can be easily measured. You can also determine whether your levels are too low by assessing your symptoms.

Measuring Progesterone

Most people are accustomed to taking traditional blood tests for measuring progesterone.

But Dr. Lee believed traditional blood tests shouldn't be used when measuring progesterone, because they don't accurately measure *biologically active* progesterone.

Biologically active progesterone is progesterone that has been absorbed by your cells and tissues. It's when progesterone is biologically active that it causes all of the wonderful changes that benefit your health.

Dr. Lee recommended saliva tests and blood spot tests as the best and most accurate tests for measuring active progesterone.

In a saliva test, you deposit saliva from your mouth into a tube. Collection can take several minutes. The tube is then sent off to the lab for analysis. In a blood spot test, your finger is pricked and the blood sample is sent to the lab for analysis.

Once your saliva or blood spot sample is analyzed, the results are sent to your doctor. He or she then can prescribe appropriate treatment based on your results.

Saliva and blood spot testing are useful for measuring mild to moderate progesterone deficiencies. When you have an extreme deficiency, it's best to be treated based upon your symptoms. Any testing you undergo will be at the discretion of your doctor.

For more information on saliva or blood spot testing, or to find a health care professional who provides them, you can contact ZRT Laboratory.

ZRT Laboratory is a lead hormone testing facility. It provides testing services worldwide through partnerships with over 9,000 healthcare professionals.

ZRT Laboratory
8605 SW Creekside Place
Beaverton, OR 97008
Phone: (503) 466-2445
Toll free: (866) 600-1636
Website: *www.zrtlab.com*
Email: *info@zrtlab.com*

Progesterone and Estrogen Must Be Measured Together

When you measure progesterone, you must measure estrogen too. Why? Because hormone balance is not based on a single amount of a particular hormone. It is based on the ratio of one hormone to another.

When trying to determine whether or not your body has enough progesterone, you need to see how much progesterone is present in relation to estrogen. The specific type of estrogen you will be measuring is estradiol (E2).

Dr. Lee stated that a healthy saliva progesterone-to-estradiol ratio for men and women is 200 to 300 to 1.

Symptoms-Based Treatment

A saliva or blood spot test is not the only way to determine if your body needs more progesterone. As we mentioned earlier, you can assess your symptoms too.

On the next page is a list of symptoms and disorders that can develop in your body when it's not making enough progesterone. This is the list I read when I discovered I had a progesterone deficiency.

Some of the disorders are present only in women; others are present in women and men.

SYMPTOMS AND DISORDERS ASSOCIATED WITH LOW PROGESTERONE LEVELS INCLUDE:

- Acceleration of the aging process
- Allergies, including asthma, rashes, sinus congestion
- Autoimmune disorders such as lupus erythematosus and thyroiditis
- Breast tenderness
- Cervical dysplasia
- Cold hands and feet, relating to thyroid dysfunction
- Copper excess
- Decreased sex drive
- Depression with anxiety or agitation
- Dry eyes
- Early onset of menstruation
- Endometrial (uterine) cancer
- Fat gain, especially around the abdomen, hips, and thighs
- Fatigue
- Fibrocystic breasts
- Foggy thinking
- Gallbladder disease
- Hair loss
- Headaches
- Hypoglycemia
- Increased blood clotting (increasing risk of strokes)
- Infertility
- Irregular menstrual periods
- Irritability
- Insomnia
- Magnesium deficiency
- Memory loss
- Miscarriage
- Mood swings
- Osteoporosis
- Polycystic ovaries
- Premenopausal bone loss
- PMS
- Prostate cancer
- Sluggish metabolism
- Thyroid dysfunction mimicking hypothyroidism
- Uterine cancer
- Uterine fibroids
- Water retention, bloating
- Zinc deficiency

Reprinted by permission from The Official Web Site of Dr. John R. Lee, M.D. (www.JohnLeeMD.com)

If you are experiencing many of the symptoms on this list, you may be able to get treated based on this. However, you will need to go to a doctor who has experience correcting these types of imbalances.

Information on how to find such a doctor will be provided later in this book.

Make sure that you discuss any symptoms that you are experiencing with a licensed medical professional.

RULE 2: TAKE BIOIDENTICAL PROGESTERONE INSTEAD OF SYNTHETIC PROGESTINS

Once it has been determined that you need progesterone — whether based on testing or your symptoms — you will need to know what kind of progesterone to take.

There are two types of progesterone you may choose from. One type, *bio-identical progesterone*, is identical to the hormone made by your body. The other, *progestin*, is not.

When you need to supplement your body with progesterone, you should only take bioidentical progesterone.

Bioidentical Progesterone

Bioidentical progesterone can do all of the things in your body that you need it to do because it is an exact replica of the progesterone made by the body.

Bioidentical progesterone can heal your brain and adrenal glands because the body accepts bioidentical progesterone as if it had made the hormone itself.

Below is an image of a progesterone molecule made by the body (endogenous), and an image of a lab-created bioidentical progesterone molecule.

PROGESTERONE MADE BY THE BODY

LAB-CREATED BIOIDENTICAL PROGESTERONE

As you can see, the two molecules look exactly the same.

When your body is not able to make the progesterone it needs on its own, bioidentical progesterone is the next best thing.

Progestins

Progestins are sort of, but not quite, like progesterone. As such, they can't do all of the things you need them to do. Progestins don't heal the brain or adrenal glands. And they may cause more harm than good.

Some of the side effects associated with using progestins include nausea, jaundice, depression, insomnia, headache, nervousness, vomiting, leg cramps, worsening of asthma and epilepsy, and changes in libido.

Progestins are commonly used in birth control and as a part of hormone replacement therapy (HRT). The most commonly prescribed progestin is medroxyprogesterone acetate (Provera).

Below is an image of the progesterone molecule made by the body, and an image of the progestin medroxyprogesterone acetate.

PROGESTERONE MADE BY THE BODY

MEDROXYPROGESTERONE ACETATE (PROVERA)

As you can see the two are not the same.

If you notice a difference between the two molecules, so will your brain.

There is no reason to use a progestin, when bioidentical progesterone is readily available.

How can I obtain bioidentical progesterone?

There are two ways to get bioidentical progesterone. You can buy it over the counter (e.g., without a prescription) at your local health food store or online. You can also get it from a compounding pharmacy with a prescription from your doctor.

Either way, you should be sure it comes in the transdermal form, has at least 450-500 milligrams (mg) of progesterone per ounce, and has progesterone as its only active ingredient.

Transdermal Progesterone

Transdermal progesterone is progesterone that has been prepared to be delivered through the skin. Most transdermal progesterone products come in a cream or gel base. You apply it in the same way that you do with lotion —you simply rub it in. Then it's absorbed and delivered to all of the places where it is needed.

Most people are accustomed to taking supplements or hormones by mouth, but Dr. Lee preferred transdermal progesterone over oral progesterone. Why?

Transdermal progesterone isn't destroyed by digestion the way oral progesterone is.

If you take 20 mg of progesterone transdermally, your body will use all 20 mg of it.

If you take 20 mg of progesterone orally, the bulk of it will be destroyed by your liver and your body must use what's left over.

Consequently, oral doses have to be 10 to 20 times higher than transdermal doses to offset what is broken down by the liver.

Dr. Lee believed that taking progesterone orally puts too much stress on your liver, causing unnatural breakdown products. All of this can be avoided by taking progesterone transdermally.

Almost all over-the-counter products come in the transdermal form. If you are going to be taking progesterone orally, you will need a prescription from your doctor.

Tips on Using Progesterone Cream

- Make sure that you apply your cream on thin-skinned areas such as your inner arms, face, or neck.
- Make sure that you apply the cream to different areas so that it can be better absorbed.
- Never apply progesterone cream before taking a bath or shower. You should always use progesterone cream after your bath or shower, giving the cream the opportunity to be absorbed.
- You can divide your dose in half. You can take a portion of your cream in the morning and then another portion before you go to bed at night.
- Progesterone has a calming effect on the body, so you may find it helpful to take your larger dose at bedtime.

How long does it take for progesterone cream to work?

Transdermal progesterone begins circulating in the blood mere seconds after it's applied. It reaches its peak in about 3 to 4 hours and its levels begin dropping after about 8 hours. Most progesterone is cleared from the body 12 hours after it's applied.

Why must creams contain at least 450-500 mg of progesterone per ounce?

Creams containing 450-500 mg of progesterone per ounce are able to deliver doses that are therapeutic to the body (20- 25 mg per ¼ teaspoon application). These amounts will make more sense when we go over dosages.

Why should progesterone be the only active ingredient in products I use?

It is very difficult to discern the effects of progesterone in your body if you are using a product that has more than one active ingredient.

By using a cream that has only progesterone as its active ingredient, you will be able to feel the impact that progesterone alone is having on your body.

There will also be times when you will need to increase your dose of progesterone. If you have a cream with another active ingredient, you will not be able to increase your progesterone dose without increasing the amount of the other ingredient.

Over-the-Counter Creams

There are lots of companies that make progesterone creams. Some companies make creams according to Dr. Lee's specifications and some of them do not.

BELOW IS A LIST OF COMPANIES THAT MAKE TRANSDERMAL CREAMS ACCORDING TO DR. LEE'S SPECIFICATIONS.

John Lee M.D. Solutions
Phone: (714) 375-3363 (outside the United States)
Toll free: (877) 375-3363
www.progesterall.com
They make *ProgesterAll* cream. This company is owned by the family of Dr. Lee.

Emerita
Phone: (503)226-1010
Toll free: (800) 888-6041
www.emerita.com
They make *Pro-Gest*—the original natural progesterone cream. Dr. Lee used Pro-Gest in his practice.

Kevala, a division of Karuna
Toll free: (888) 749-8643
www.kevalahealth.com
Makers of *PureGest* cream. PureGest is free of additional hormones, herbs and alcohol.

Life-flo Health Care Products
Toll free: (888) 999-7440
www.life-flo.com
They make *Progesta-Care* cream.

Dr. Randolph's Natural Balance Cream
Toll free: (866) 628-6337
www.hormonewell.com
Dr. Randolph's Natural Balance Cream contains only progesterone as its active ingredient, and no chemicals.

This is not a complete listing.

If you find a cream that you would like to use that is not found on this list, check with the cream's manufacturer to be certain the cream contains at least 450-500 mg of progesterone per ounce, and that progesterone is the only active ingredient in the product.

Make sure to consult a licensed medical professional before using any over-the-counter product.

Progesterone by Prescription

Traditionally, prescriptions for bioidentical progesterone had to be filled at compounding pharmacies. But because bioidentical hormones are in such high demand now, some chain pharmacies are starting to prepare them as well.

If you have a prescription for bioidentical progesterone, call your local drug store to see if it can fill your prescription. If not, you will need to take your prescription to your local compounding pharmacy.

Compounding pharmacies, like commercial drug stores, are regulated by their particular state's pharmacy licensing board. They are able to provide many services that aren't offered at most drug stores.

Compounding pharmacies can combine several prescriptions into one. They can add flavor additives to children's prescriptions, and they can prepare a wide variety of bioidentical hormones, including bioidentical progesterone.

To find the compounding pharmacy nearest you, contact the International Academy of Compounding Pharmacists (IACP) toll free at (800) 927-4227 or go online at *www.iacprx.org* and click on the "find a compounding pharmacist" link.

If you would like more information on pharmacy compounding, you can visit the website *www.compoundingfacts.org*.

Your Prescription Must Be for Bioidentical Progesterone

When your doctor writes you a prescription for progesterone, the prescription must be written for "bioidentical progesterone." Your doctor cannot write a prescription for a progestin and expect the pharmacy to convert it to whatever form you would like.

If your doctor is unfamiliar with prescribing bioidentical progesterone, but is willing to prescribe it for you, put him or her in touch with your local compounding pharmacy.

The Different Preparations of Progesterone

Progesterone can be prepared in many different strengths (greater than 500 mg per ounce) and forms (transdermally, orally, or by injection).

Over-the-counter preparations usually contain no more than 550 mg per ounce and usually come only in the transdermal form.

According to Dr. Lee, the only time you will need a cream that contains more than 500 mg of progesterone per ounce is when you are first balancing your hormones and trying to restore depleted levels.

Once your levels are restored, creams containing 450-500 mg per ounce are sufficient for most people.

How is bioidentical progesterone made?

To appreciate how bioidentical progesterone is made, you must understand how the body makes progesterone.

The body makes progesterone from cholesterol. Scientists aren't able to convert human cholesterol into progesterone yet, but they are able to convert cholesterol-like substances found in certain plants into progesterone. These substances are called *saponins*.

Using a simple process, scientists convert plant saponins into real, identical to the body progesterone.

How are progestins made?

Most progestins are made from plant sources like bioidentical progesterone. Their manufacturers intentionally make them different from the progesterone the body makes so they can be patented as unique substances. Patented progestins are great for business, but they are toxic to the body.

RULE 3: TAKE PROGESTERONE IN PHYSIOLOGICAL AMOUNTS ONLY

Once it's been determined you need progesterone and you know what kind of progesterone you are going to take, you will need to know how *much* to take.

Figuring it out is simple. Dr. Lee cautioned when taking progesterone, you should only take the amount that your body would be making if it were healthy—in other words, a physiological amount.

Dr. Lee established guidelines on how to take progesterone. His recommendations are found in the table on the next page.

In a Nutshell-Transdermal Progesterone
When and How Much

(Note: These doses are for transdermal progesterone, e.g., creams, gels, and oils.) Getting each dab of cream to be exactly right size isn't critical, because there's a buffering effect as the progesterone is absorbed into subcutaneous (under the skin) fat. The release of the hormone from body fat serves to make the progesterone effect relatively steady even if daily doses vary a little.

Premenopausal (having menstrual cycles): 20 to 30 mg progesterone for the two weeks before menstruation begins.

Menopausal (not having menstrual cycles): 10 to 20 mg of progesterone daily in divided doses (e.g., 5 to 10 mg twice daily) for 24 to 26 consecutive days a month, stopping four to five days each month.

Men: 8 to 10 mg of progesterone for 24 to 26 consecutive days a month, stopping for four to five days each month.*

From DR. JOHN LEE'S HORMONE BALANCE MADE SIMPLE by VIRGINIA HOPKINS. Copyright © 2006 by the Estate of John R. Lee, M.D. and Virginia Hopkins. By permissions of GRAND CENTRAL PUBLISHING.
*Reprinted by permission from The Official Web Site of Dr. John R. Lee, M.D. (www.JohnLeeMD.com).

The recommendations in the table are based on the transdermal application of progesterone.

If you are going to take progesterone orally, the amounts you will need will be higher than the amounts in the table.

Before You Start

If you have developed bipolar disorder or schizophrenia, it means your body has been functioning without sufficient progesterone for many years.

In this case, before you start taking amounts recommended by Dr. Lee, you will need to catch up by taking a *loading dose*. A loading dose is a larger-than-normal dose used to restore depleted levels. It is recommended for people with severely low progesterone levels.

A loading dose can be five times or more the amounts in Dr. Lee's table.

Your doctor will help you to find a loading dose that's right for you. Once your progesterone levels are restored, you will begin to take amounts that are similar to the ones found in the table.

How long will I need to take loading doses?

There is no special timetable for taking a loading dose. Hormone balance is an individualized endeavor. What's good for you may not be good for someone else. One person may need to take a loading dose for the first two months; someone else may need to take higher doses for the first four.

I took higher doses for the first four months, but that doesn't mean that you will have to. When taking progesterone, always use your symptoms as your guide.

Are you still having mood swings or hearing voices? Are you crying uncontrollably? In other words, are you still having symptoms of mental disease?

As long as you are experiencing symptoms of mental illness, your body doesn't have the progesterone it needs. So you will need to continue to take larger doses.

As your symptoms improve, your loading dose can be decreased to amounts similar to the ones found in Dr. Lee's table.

5
RECOVERY STEP-BY-STEP

Now that you know the basics of taking progesterone, let's go over the different issues that can arise when balancing your hormones.

In this chapter, we will look at the different issues men and women may face. Some women want to know if they can take progesterone while taking birth control pills or hormone replacement therapy (HRT). Some men want to know if progesterone will have feminizing affects on them.

We will also go over what recovery will entail for each group.

Recovery for Premenopausal Women

If you are premenopausal (still having menstrual cycles), Dr. Lee recommended that you take 20-30 mg of progesterone a day during the two weeks before the first day of your period.

This dose will mimic what healthy premenopausal women's bodies do.

Because your progesterone supplementation is built around your menstrual cycle, you will need to use a calendar to figure out the days you will take progesterone.

	1	2	3	4	5	6
7	8	9	10	11	12	13
14	15	16	17	18	19	20
21	22	23	24	25	26	27
28	29	30	31			

Using the calendar, circle the first day of your period and then count back two weeks from that date.

These are the dates you will be taking progesterone.

Write your dates below:
I will need to take 20-30 mg of progesterone from the _____ to the _____ of every month.

When taking progesterone, you should always stop a day or two before your expected period. By doing so, you will allow your body to have its monthly cycle. It is the fall of estrogen and progesterone that causes the monthly menstrual cycle.

Make sure you always use a calendar to keep track of the days when you are supposed to take progesterone. You may be tempted to rely on your memory, but this is not advisable. It is very easy to miss a dose if you do that.

The Importance of a Loading Dose for Premenopausal Women

Remember: when you first start taking progesterone, you will need to take loading doses to restore depleted levels. Your loading dose will be timed around your menstrual cycle.

For your loading dose, you will be taking higher amounts of progesterone for the three weeks you are not on your menstrual cycle.

Then you take one week off to allow for your monthly cycle.

Once your hormones become balanced and your symptoms improve, you will only take progesterone for the two weeks before menstruation begins.

Special Issues for Premenopausal Women

Now that you know how to take progesterone, let's go over some of the issues that you may face as a premenopausal woman.

The most common issues are regarding birth control pills and irregular menstrual cycles.

If You Are Taking Birth Control Pills:

You should not take birth control pills and progesterone at the same time.

Most birth control pills contain synthetic estrogens and progestins. If you take progesterone along with these substances, it will be very difficult to determine what effect each chemical is having on your body, and you will have a hard time adjusting your progesterone dose.

If you are taking birth control pills for the purpose of preventing pregnancy, but you want to take progesterone, then you will need to discuss an alternative, non-hormonal birth control method with your doctor.

Once you have an alternative birth control method in place, you can start taking progesterone according to Dr. Lee's specifications. Taking progesterone alone will not prevent pregnancy.

If you are taking birth control pills for the sole purpose of correcting an irregular cycle, taking progesterone alone will also do the job.

If You Have Irregular Periods:

Whether you have an irregular period that comes on a different day every month, one that comes every other month, or one that comes only once or twice a year, you can still figure out when to take progesterone.

If you have a period that comes on different days every month, you can use the date of your last period to determine when you will need to take progesterone. You will count back two weeks from this date. This will be the time frame that you will need to take progesterone.

Make sure that you use a calendar to keep track of your dates.

If you can't remember the date of your last period, you can start taking progesterone (20-30 mg) from the 1st of every month until the 14th of every month. Your period should then start on or around the 15th of every month.

If you have never had a regular menstrual cycle before, taking progesterone should stabilize your cycles.

Taking progesterone alone has been approved by the Food and Drug Administration (FDA) for the treatment of amenorrhea (absent menstrual cycles).

Issues of Using Progesterone for Premenopausal Women

- Taking progesterone can alter the days of your menstrual cycle
- You might experience breakthrough bleeding until you figure out your proper doses

As you get a handle on your timing, these issues should be resolved over time.

Many women (me included) say that the benefits of using progesterone outweigh the minor mishaps that can occur in the initial stages of supplementation.

Make sure you discuss any symptoms that you are experiencing with your doctor.

The Benefits of Using Progesterone for Premenopausal Women

PROGESTERONE:
- Stabilizes moods
- Helps normalize blood sugar levels
- Stabilizes irregular menstrual cycles
- Eliminates hormone-related migraine headaches
- Improves sleep
- Reduces and sometimes eliminates painful symptoms associated with endometriosis
- Eliminates breast fibrocysts
- Improves and sometimes eliminates symptoms of premenstrual syndrome (PMS) and premenstrual dysphoric disorder (PMDD)

For more information on how progesterone can help you, read *Dr. John Lee's Hormone Balance Made Simple* (Wellness Central, 2006).

Recovery for Menopausal Women

Progesterone supplementation is pretty straightforward for you. According to Dr. Lee, you should take 10-20 mg of progesterone for 24-26 consecutive days a month.

The easiest way to keep track is to take progesterone starting on the 1st of every month and then stop on the 24th- 26th of every month.

When you first start taking progesterone, you will need to take larger doses for the first couple of months until your symptoms improve. Then, you will be able to take the recommended 10-20 mg of progesterone per day.

For some women, this regimen will be enough. But if you're taking hormone replacement therapy (HRT) or if you've had one or both of your ovaries removed, you may want to know what taking progesterone means for you.

Let's go through each scenario, one by one.

If You Are on Hormone Replacement Therapy:

Hormone replacement therapy (HRT) usually consists of a synthetic estrogen and/or progestin. These synthetic hormones are typically meant to replace the hormones that are loss during a hysterectomy. Sometimes a doctor prescribes HRT for a woman who has entered menopause.

If you are taking HRT, you can still take progesterone.

However, if the HRT you are taking consists of a synthetic estrogen and progestin, Dr. Lee recommended that you stop taking your progestin and switch to bioidentical progesterone. He also recommended that you wean yourself from estrogen.

To switch to bioidentical progesterone, you can buy an over-the-counter cream or else ask the same doctor who prescribed your progestin to write you a prescription for the bioidentical kind. Remember, you can put your doctor in touch with your local compounding pharmacy if your doctor is unfamiliar with prescribing bioidentical progesterone.

Once you have made the switch, you will be able to be weaned off of your estrogen.

There are two ways to do this: (1) You can reduce your estrogen intake by 50% by taking your estrogen pill every other day for 24 days, then take the rest of the month off; or (2) you can ask the doctor who prescribed your estrogen to put you on a lower dose. Dr. Lee says that you can continue to lower your dose every 2 to 3 months, until you are completely weaned off.

Never stop taking estrogen suddenly. Always gradually reduce your dose. Otherwise, Dr. Lee warned, you could develop menopausal symptoms like hot flashes and vaginal dryness.

Make sure to consult a licensed medical professional if you would like to make changes to your hormone replacement therapy.

I thought all menopausal women needed estrogen. Shouldn't I take estrogen if I've had my ovaries removed?

Once upon a time doctors were taught that estrogen went to zero at menopause, but Dr. Lee felt this is not true. Rather, he said, it is only reduced by 40%- 60%—even if a woman has had her ovaries removed.

Dr. Lee explained that menopausal women can make estrogen from their body fat, when their ovaries are not able to make enough.

The body fat converts the adrenal hormone, androstenedione, into estrogen.

A menopausal woman with a high percentage of body fat makes more estrogen than a premenopausal woman who has low amounts of body fat.

So if you are going through menopause this does not mean that you automatically need estrogen, even if you have had your ovaries removed.

If you are experiencing symptoms of bipolar disorder and schizophrenia, you definitely don't need more estrogen. Symptoms of mental illness are caused by the body not making enough progesterone to balance the effects of estrogen.

If you are taking estrogen and are having symptoms of mental illness, there is a good chance that the estrogen you are taking is making your current symptoms worse.

Measure Testosterone Too

If you've had a hysterectomy, there is a good chance your testosterone levels are low too. Testosterone is a "male" hormone, but women also make it in small amounts for sex drive (libido) and bone health. If your body isn't making the testosterone it needs, you may experience memory or bone loss, fatigue, or low libido.

If you suspect your testosterone levels are low, you can check your levels via a saliva test. If you're deficient, it can be treated by taking 0.1 to 1 mg of transdermal (creams, gels) testosterone daily or every other day.

Like progesterone, it's best to take testosterone transdermally, in its bioidentical form. Testosterone is available only by prescription.

Issues of Using Progesterone for Menopausal Women

You may experience vaginal bleeding or spotting when you start progesterone. Don't worry, this doesn't mean your menstrual cycle has started again.

The bleeding from taking progesterone is caused by the shedding of your uterine lining; it has probably been building up for months or years from excessive estrogen in your body.

Once your hormones are within healthy, physiological levels and the lining is fully shed, you shouldn't experience any more breakthrough bleeding.

The Benefits of Using Progesterone for Menopausal Women

PROGESTERONE:

- Stabilizes moods
- Helps to build new bone, reversing osteoporosis
- Eliminates water retention and swelling associated with a hormonal imbalance
- Improves muscle aches and pains
- Improves clarity of thinking
- Hydrates skin
- Stabilizes sleep

In order to learn more about how progesterone can improve your health, read *Dr. John Lee's Hormone Balance Made Simple* (Wellness Central, 2006) and *What Your Doctor May Not Tell You About Menopause* (Wellness Central, 2004).

Recovery for Men

Progesterone supplementation is clear-cut for you. Dr. Lee says you will need to take 8-10 mg of progesterone for 24-26 consecutive days a month. The easiest way to keep track is to take progesterone from the 1st to the 24th or 26th of every month and then take the rest of the month off.

When you first start taking progesterone, you will need to take larger doses so that your body can compensate for all of the years it hasn't been making sufficient progesterone. As your symptoms improve, your loading dose can be decreased to physiological doses of 8-10 mg. You should always work with a doctor in finding your right dose.

Will taking progesterone cause me to develop female characteristics?

Progesterone does not cause feminizing characteristics in men or women. Estrogen and testosterone are the hormones that cause sexual characteristics, not progesterone.

High levels of estrogen will cause breast development in men or women, just as high testosterone levels will cause an increase in body hair and voice deepening in men or women.

Progesterone causes no such effects. It balances the effects of estrogen.

Part of the confusion surrounding progesterone occurred when the hormone was first discovered. Doctors learned it was necessary for pregnancy. Since only women can become pregnant, it was assumed that only women needed it. This could not be further from the truth.

Men and women both need progesterone for their mental and physical health.

The Benefits of Using Progesterone for Men

PROGESTERONE:
- Stabilizes moods
- Improves sleep
- Reduces anxiety
- Increases energy levels
- Improves digestion
- Reduces the risk of prostate cancer

There aren't very many books written on the topic of hormone balance for men, but hopefully this will soon change.

Two books that are available for you to read are Dr. Lee's 28-page booklet *Hormone Balance for Men* (Hormones Etc., 2003) and Dr. Eugene Shippen's *The Testosterone Syndrome* (M. Evans and Company, 2001).

Dr. Lee's *Hormone Balance for Men* was written primarily for doctors, but it contains good information for the interested layperson as well, including progesterone's role in prostate health.

Dr. Shippen's *The Testosterone Syndrome* shows how hormones are essential to male health. Dr. Shippen doesn't focus on progesterone, but he discusses how hormones influence your health in general.

What Men and Women Can Expect When Taking Progesterone

When you first start taking progesterone, you may feel a little worse before you feel better. In fact, you should expect to experience a temporary worsening in your symptoms.

Why? Dr. Lee says that when estrogen has been present in your body for a long time unopposed (unbalanced) by progesterone, the estrogen receptors in your body tune down.

When progesterone is finally introduced to the body, the receptors come back to full strength—causing symptoms associated with high estrogen levels. In other words, your symptoms can become more intense or you may develop some new ones.

This is temporary. As your body begins to rid itself of excessive estrogen and your progesterone levels are restored, you should not experience these symptoms again.

How long will it take for me to notice an improvement in my symptoms?

Once you've started taking progesterone along with the proper loading doses, you should notice an improvement in symptoms within 3 to 4 weeks. Remember, though, this is just an estimate.

How long will it take for me to experience a full recovery?

It can take several months to correct a severe progesterone deficiency. Taking progesterone will not make your symptoms go away overnight. Instead, you should notice a gradual improvement in your symptoms over time, until they disappear. One person may experience a full recovery within 6 months; for another person, recovery may take a year or longer. Once your symptoms are eliminated, you will need to continue taking progesterone to maintain your health.

Can I take progesterone if I am taking psychiatric medications?

If you are currently taking psychiatric medications, continue to take them as prescribed, and work on balancing your hormones at the same time.

You cannot wean yourself off of your psychiatric medications. Only your prescribing doctor can do this. There are serious side effects that can occur if you try to do it yourself.

Make sure that you tell your prescribing doctor that you will be balancing your hormones and that you would like to be weaned off your medications accordingly.

Putting It All Together

There is no special formula for hormone balance. There is no "one size fits all" therapy. Every *body* is different. You will need to work with your doctor to find a regimen that will work for you.

However, even though everyone will have specialized treatment, the core principles are the same. Remember:

- You Should Take Progesterone Only if You Need It
- Use Bioidentical Progesterone Instead of Synthetic Progestins
- Take Progesterone in Normal, Physiological Amounts Only

If you stick to these rules and work with a doctor who understands these rules, you will be well on your way toward recovery.

You can also help your body along by having a support group (this group can consist of family and friends), getting plenty of rest, engaging in some type of physical activity, eating a healthy diet that includes a large variety of fruits and vegetables, and by doing things you enjoy and avoiding things that stress you out.

6
FINDING A DOCTOR

The key to your recovery is finding the right doctor to work with. If you have heart problems, you go to a cardiologist. If you have foot problems, you go to a podiatrist. When you are having progesterone problems, you need to go to a doctor who specializes in hormone balance.

But here's the problem: there is no such thing as a hormone balance doctor. There are many types of doctors from which you must choose.

Some are gynecologists. Others are internists, family doctors, or endocrinologists. When selecting your doctor you should not focus on the specialty. Instead, your focus should be on the type of service a doctor can provide.

If you are taking birth control pills or hormone replacement therapy, you will need to work with a doctor who has experience with these issues. This could be a family doctor or gynecologist.

If you are male, you will need to work with a doctor who has experience treating men with hormonal imbalances.

Using Your Local Pharmacy

One of the best ways to find the right doctor is to contact your local compounding pharmacy. Most compounding pharmacies keep a list of associated doctors and many of them are happy to make referrals.

Ask your compounding specialist to refer you to a doctor who has experience prescribing progesterone and treating patients with mood disorders.

To find the compounding pharmacy nearest you, contact the International Academy of Compounding Pharmacists (IACP) toll free at (800) 927-4227 or online at *www.iacprx.org*.

You can also search your local yellow pages to find a doctor, or online at *www.yellowpages.com*.

Many doctors who specialize in hormone balance advertise under the labels of preventative, anti-aging, alternative, or holistic medicine.

You can also find a medical professional by contacting the organizations below:

ZRT Laboratory
8605 SW Creekside Place
Beaverton, OR 97008
Phone: (503) 466-2445
Toll free: (866) 600-1636
Website: *www.zrtlab.com*
Email: *info@zrtlab.com*

American Association of Naturopathic Physicians
4435 Wisconsin Avenue, NW, Suite 403
Washington, DC 20016
Phone: (202) 237-8150
Toll free: (866) 538-2267
Website: *www.naturopathic.org*
Email: *member.services@naturopathic.org*

American College for Advancement in Medicine
8001 Irvine Center Drive, Suite 825
Irvine, CA 92618
Toll free: (800) 532-3688
Website: *www.acam.org*
Email: *info@acam.org*

American Holistic Medical Association
23366 Commerce Park, Suite 101B
Beachwood, OH 44122
Phone: (216) 292-6644
Website: *www.holisticmedicine.org*
Email: *info@holisticmedicine.org*

American Osteopathic Association
142 East Ontario Street
Chicago, IL 60611
Phone: (312) 202-8000
Toll free: (800) 621-1773
Website: *www.osteopathic.org*
Email: *msc@osteopathic.org*

Make sure you work with a licensed medical professional in balancing your hormones. Progesterone is sold over the counter, but this is not an imbalance you should attempt to correct yourself. You should always be under the care of a licensed medical professional.

Information for Doctors

If you are a doctor who is interested in incorporating hormone balance into your practice, you can contact the Dr. John Lee Institute at:

619 Madison Street, Suite 100
Oregon City, OR 97045
Phone: (503) 342-8380
Website: *www.drjohnleeinstitute.com*

The Dr. John Lee Institute (DJLI) educates healthcare providers in the art and science of natural hormone balancing.

The Institute is accredited by the Accreditation Council for Continuing Medical Education (ACCME) to provide continuing medical education for physicians.

7
QUESTIONS AND ANSWERS

Q: IF PROGESTERONE IS SO GREAT, WHY HASN'T MY PSYCHIATRIST TOLD ME ABOUT IT?

A: Your psychiatrist hasn't told you about progesterone yet because he or she doesn't know its benefits. Hormone balance isn't taught during psychiatry residency training.

Dr. Lee noted that medical school is like a trade school. He was taught that if a patient had hypertension he was to give them a diuretic (water pill), but not much was done to address where the hypertension was coming from.

Doctors are trained to treat the symptoms of diseases, but not much study is done in terms of preventing them.

And this is the case with psychiatry. Psychiatrists are taught to prescribe medications (antidepressants, antipsychotics, and mood stabilizers) according to one's symptoms, but they aren't taught how to correct the underlying causes. Hopefully this will soon change.

Q: MY PSYCHIATRIC MEDICATIONS WORK SO WELL. WHY SHOULD I ALTER MY TREATMENT TO TRY PROGESTERONE?

A: The most effective psychiatric medications work by influencing the secretion of progesterone. So if your medications are only working because they are increasing your progesterone levels, wouldn't it be better to take progesterone instead?

Even if your psychiatric medications offer some relief from your symptoms, they can never stop or correct the physical deterioration that can result from low progesterone.

Psychiatric medications can't build new bone. They can't correct hormone-related fatigue, and they can't improve hormone-related digestive or thyroid disorders. In other words, psychiatric medications can never do what progesterone does.

If your body is not making enough progesterone, you will need to give it progesterone to experience optimal health.

Q: I HAVE A LOVED ONE WHO IS REALLY SICK AND I THINK THEY WOULD BENEFIT FROM HAVING THEIR HORMONES BALANCED. HOW CAN I CONVINCE SOMEONE TO TAKE PROGESTERONE, WHEN THEY DON'T BELIEVE THEY ARE SICK?

A: It can be very difficult to convince someone with a mental illness that they have an illness, because the illness can interfere with one's ability to be rational or think logically.

If you have a family member is who not aware of their illness, you can still help them.

You can suggest progesterone to your family member for the treatment of any of the physical symptoms that Dr. Lee has associated with low progesterone levels. Does your loved one suffer from migraine headaches, fatigue, or a digestive disorder? Then, you may be able to convince your loved one to seek treatment for one of these symptoms — and see what else clears up.

Q: ARE THERE ANY SIDE EFFECTS ASSOCIATED WITH USING BIOIDENTICAL PROGESTERONE?

A: Dr. Lee says that there are no side effects associated with using bioidentical progesterone if using the correct physiological amounts (the amounts the body makes when it's healthy).

However, if you take too much progesterone or more than what your body needs, you might experience symptoms like drowsiness, water retention, mild depression, bloating, lowered libido, candida, and sleepiness. The key to hormone supplementation is balance. Too little progesterone can be detrimental to your health and so can too much.

Q: WILL TAKING PROGESTERONE HELP ME FEEL PERFECT ALL THE TIME?

A: I wondered the same thing, but progesterone can't make you feel perfect. If you lose a loved one, you will experience sadness. If you stay awake all night, you will be fatigued. Progesterone can't stop life from happening to you. But it can correct hormone-related sadness and fatigue and it can make navigating through life easier by stabilizing your moods and mind.

Q: ARE MENTAL ILLNESSES INHERITED?
A: Absolutely yes.

You resemble your parents from the inside out. This is why you have to complete a family medical history questionnaire whenever you visit your doctor. Your doctor wants to know what health issues your relatives have, because certain medical conditions can be passed from parent to child. And progesterone deficiencies are one of these conditions.

Progesterone deficiencies can take on many different manifestations. Everyone in your family doesn't have to have bipolar disorder or schizophrenia.

One person in your family might have clinical depression, while someone else may have an attention deficit disorder, anxiety, or thyroid disorder or an autoimmune disease.

There are so many illnesses that can stem from a progesterone deficiency, because progesterone impacts so many systems in the body.

Q: HOW IS IT THAT ONE HORMONE CAN BE USED FOR PREGNANCY AND YET THE SAME HORMONE IS ALSO ESSENTIAL FOR BRAIN FUNCTIONING?
A: That's the beauty of the body. Progesterone has multiple effects in the body because of DNA, the genetic information stored inside cells.

When progesterone acts on your cells, it unlocks that genetic information and causes them to perform various functions. When progesterone acts on cells in the uterine lining, the lining thickens. When progesterone acts on your brain cells, your brain can process information clearly.

Q: I DEVELOPED SYMPTOMS OF MENTAL ILLNESS AFTER A HEAD INJURY; WILL TAKING PROGESTERONE HELP ME TOO?
A: Anything that interferes with your brain's ability to communicate clearly can cause symptoms. A severe head injury, brain surgery, or heavy drug use can all cause symptoms similar to ones seen in mental illness. Progesterone can reduce the severity of a head injury and reduce swelling caused by surgery. But it's not known if progesterone can reverse symptoms caused by substance abuse.

Q: CAN CHILDREN HAVE PROGESTERONE DEFICIENCIES?
A: Yes. This means children can develop mental illnesses just as adults do. Often, children with mental illnesses go undiagnosed. This is because traditionally a diagnosis of mental illness is dependent upon one's ability to recognize and report their symptoms. That can be difficult for a child to do. Even when a child is aware, they often lack the verbal ability to express what is happening to them.

Many children in the earliest stages of a progesterone deficiency are diagnosed with an attention deficit disorder, anxiety, or conduct disorder.

Children with progesterone deficiencies can also develop some of the physical symptoms identified by Dr. Lee. One child may develop allergies and another child may have an overactive immune system causing swollen lymph nodes.

Q: SO HOW DO I HELP MY CHILD? CAN MY CHILD TAKE PROGESTERONE TOO?
A: Children who have mental illnesses are often prescribed psychiatric drugs, just as if they were adults. Dr. Michael Platt is the only doctor I know of who has used progesterone to treat children with attention, emotional, and behavioral disorders.

Dr. Platt is an internist based in Rancho Mirage, California. He explained in his book, *The Miracle of Bioidentical Hormones* (Clancy Lane Publishing, 2007), that he uses progesterone to treat children only when he knows that one of the child's parents has an imbalance.

What Dr. Platt is doing is not the norm—even though it should be. New research needs to be done in the field of hormonal balance in children. Progesterone ranges need to be established for children, so that those with progesterone deficiencies can be treated.

Giving hormones to children isn't as controversial as it sounds. Juvenile diabetes is treated by giving children insulin. No one would make a child with diabetes wait until their 18th birthday before they could start taking insulin if their body wasn't making enough of it.

Progesterone needs to be viewed in the same light. Would you make a child wait until their 18th birthday before they could start taking progesterone, even if you knew their body wasn't making enough of it? Of course not. That would be inhumane and illegal.

The sooner progesterone ranges can be established for children, the sooner the lives of progesterone-deficient children can be improved.

If progesterone deficiencies are caught in their earliest stages, many cases of mental illness can be prevented. Thus many children would be spared the pain and stigma that can come from living with mental disease.

Q: I PREFER TO TAKE PROGESTERONE ORALLY (IN PILLS AND CAPSULES). HOW DO I OBTAIN IT?

A: Progesterone capsules are sold commercially under the trade name Prometrium. It's available in strengths of 100 mg and 200 mg. The progesterone in Prometrium is dissolved in peanut oil, so if you are allergic to peanuts you won't be able to take Prometrium.

To obtain oral progesterone without peanut oil, your doctor will need to write you a prescription for peanut oil-free progesterone capsules. A compounding pharmacist will be able to prepare it for you. Both Prometrium and peanut oil-free progesterone capsules are available only by prescription.

Q: I HEARD THAT PROGESTERONE CAUSES CANCER, IS THIS TRUE?

A: No.

If progesterone caused cancer, every human being born into the world would have cancer! During childbirth, a baby is subjected to the highest amounts of progesterone ever in its entire life. Pregnant women make about 400 mg (milligrams) of progesterone per day during their last trimester, which is well over 8 times the amount premenopausal women make after ovulation and over 20 times the amount men and menopausal women make.

Dr. Lee noted that reports of progesterone being linked to cancer are usually referring to a progestin —not progesterone.

There are still some medical professionals who are not aware that progestins and progesterone are not the same. So they make comments about progesterone being linked to cancer, when in fact they are talking about a progestin.

Progestins have been linked to cancer. Progesterone has not. Progesterone protects the body against cancer by balancing the effects of estrogen.

Q: DOES THE FOOD AND DRUG ADMINISTRATION (FDA) ACKNOWLEDGE THAT BIOIDENTICAL PROGESTERONE AND PROGESTINS ARE DIFFERENT?
A: Yes, but you aren't going to see a press release from the FDA that says bioidentical progesterone is better than progestins. But remember the saying: "Don't judge someone on what they say; judge them on what they do." This applies to the FDA.

As you know, progesterone is essential to pregnancy. When a woman has difficulty conceiving, she goes to a fertility specialist who will give her real, bioidentical progesterone.

And the FDA approves this. It would not do so if it didn't acknowledge that bioidentical progesterone and progesterone made by the body are the same.

The FDA prohibits the use of progestins in fertility treatments because progestins cause birth defects.

If progestins were identical to progesterone, the FDA would allow progestins to be used in fertility treatments.

Q: WILL I HAVE TO TAKE PROGESTERONE FOR THE REST OF MY LIFE?
A: Unless you are able to correct what is causing your body not to make enough progesterone, you will need to always provide your body with the extra progesterone it needs in order for you to be mentally and physically healthy.

Q: SO WHERE DO PROGESTERONE DEFICIENCIES COME FROM?
A: Dr. Lee says progesterone deficiencies can be caused by many things. They can be caused by estrogen-like chemicals found in the environment, called xenoestrogens. They can be caused by doctors who are prescribing estrogen inappropriately. They can come from a diet with more fat, more sugar, and more calories than you need. And they can come from the sex organs not being able to produce enough progesterone.

Q: IS THERE ANY SCIENTIFIC EVIDENCE THAT SHOWS THAT PROGESTERONE CAN REVERSE BIPOLAR DISORDER AND SCHIZOPHRENIA?
A: Yes. Dr. Lee helped to stabilize the moods of hundreds of people using progesterone during his 30 years of clinical practice. And he has helped thousands more through his books.
Dr. Michael Platt has reversed bipolar disorder in his patients using progesterone. He describes one of his cases in his book, *The Miracle of Bioidentical Hormones* (Clancy Lane Publishing, 2007).
There is also evidence in scientific journals. *The American Journal of Psychiatry* published a letter titled "Estrogen-progesterone combination: another mood stabilizer?" (Chouinard, Steinberg, & Steiner, 1987). This letter, published over 20 years ago, found that progesterone was responsible for regulating mood.
Evidence has also been found by doctors Pavel Katsel, Kenneth Davis, and Vahram Haroutunian of New York, NY; doctors Dimitri Tkachev, Michael Mimmack, Stephen Huffaker, Margaret Ryan and Sabine Bahn of Cambridge, the UK; and doctors Natalya Uranova, Victor Vostrikov, and Diana Orlovskaya of Moscow, who discovered that people with bipolar disorder and schizophrenia have damaged myelin sheaths.
Myelin is the protective coating that wraps around your brain cells. It helps your brain process information. Progesterone makes myelin.

Below is an image of a brain cell (neuron) and the progesterone-created myelin sheath.

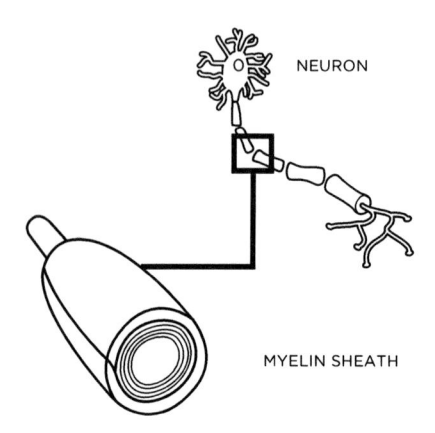

Myelin acts like an electrical cord in the brain. It helps to deliver electrical messages from one brain cell to the next.

When you have a mental illness, you have damaged myelin sheaths (because of low progesterone levels). They cause the electrical messages in your brain to misfire, creating symptoms of mental illness.

Q: IF ALL OF THIS EVIDENCE SHOWS THAT MENTAL ILLNESS IS LINKED TO LOW PROGESTERONE LEVELS, WHY DON'T DOCTORS PRESCRIBE PROGESTERONE?

A: Unfortunately, pharmaceutical companies exert powerful influence over which treatments become a part of medical practice. And pharmaceutical companies aren't interested in offering progesterone to the public because it's more profitable to treat a disease than cure it.

A year's supply of progesterone costs around $200 a year. That averages out to a little more than $16 a month for a woman. A year's supply for a man would be even less.

Psychiatric medications cost considerably more. The most expensive medications can cost up to $800 a month. And if you have more than one prescription, your monthly bill could easily top $1000. You don't have to be a mathematician to see how profitable these treatments are for pharmaceutical companies.

Q: WHAT CAN I DO TO LIMIT THE PHARAMCEUTICAL INDUSTRY'S INFLUENCE ON MEDICINE?

A: You can contact your state Congresspeople and ask them to sponsor or support bills that would prohibit drug companies from providing continuing medical education to doctors. When drug companies educate doctors, they don't discuss the latest developments in prevention—they're hawking their latest products, which may or may not be beneficial to public health.

You can also ask that drug companies be prohibited from sponsoring travel arrangements or giving gifts and other payments to physicians, because these can unfairly influence medical practice.

If you would like to contact your state senators or representative, you can find them online at *www.senate.gov* and *www.house.gov*, or you can contact them by mail or by phone by looking at the next page.

By Postal Mail

You can direct postal correspondence to your senator or to other U.S. Senate offices at the following address:

U.S. SENATORS:
Office of Senator (Name)
United States Senate
Washington, D.C. 20510

SENATE COMMITTEES:
(Name of Committee)
United States Senate
Washington, D.C. 20510

For information on how to write specific House representatives, please go to this link:
https://writerep.house.gov/writerep/welcome.shtml

By Telephone

Alternatively, you may phone the United States Capitol switchboard at (202) 224-3121. A switchboard operator will connect you directly with the Senate or Representative office you request.

CONCLUSION

"All disease comes from metabolic imbalance. When the metabolic imbalance is corrected, the disease goes away. If you fail to keep up the correction for the underlying metabolic imbalance (i.e., revert to whatever it was that created the metabolic imbalance in the first place), the disease will come back. This is called preventative medicine."

—**John R. Lee, M.D.**
Hormone Balance for Men, 2003

"Bipolar disorder and schizophrenia come from a progesterone deficiency. When the body is given the progesterone it needs, bipolar disorder and schizophrenia go away. If one were to stop taking progesterone, bipolar disorder and schizophrenia will come back. Bipolar disorder and schizophrenia are preventable diseases."

—**Doris King, CMHP**
Curing Bipolar Disorder and Schizophrenia, 2009

RESOURCES

Recommended Reading

Compounding Pharmacies

Progesterone in the UK

Finding a Doctor in the UK

References

Index

About the Author

Recommended Reading

Dr. John Lee's Hormone Balance Made Simple
(Wellness Central, 2006)

What Your Doctor May Not Tell You About Menopause
(Wellness Central, 2004)

Adrenal Fatigue: The 21st Century Stress Syndrome
(Smart Publications, 2002)

The Safe Uses of Cortisol
(Charles C. Thomas Publisher, 2004)

Natural Progesterone
(Thorsons, 2003)

Compounding Pharmacies

International Academy of Compounding Pharmacists
4638 Riverstone Blvd.
Missouri City, TX 77459
Phone: (281) 933-8400
Toll Free Referral Line: (800) 927-4227
Website: *www.iacprx.org*
Email: *iacpinfo@iacprx.org*

The Professional Compounding Centers of America (PCCA) Canada
744 Third Street
London, ON
Canada
N5V 5J2
Phone: (519) 455-0690
Toll free: (800) 668-9453
Website: *www.pccarx.ca*
Email: *customerservice@pccarx.ca*

The Professional Compounding Centers of America (PCCA) Australia
Unit 1, 73 Beauchamp Road
Matraville, NSW 2036 Australia
Phone: 02-9316-1500

Progesterone in the UK

Progesterone is a prescription only item in the UK. It can also be obtained via personal import as long as it is for your own personal use. It is illegal to import progesterone into the UK and then give it to someone else to use.

If you are interested in obtaining progesterone via import, you can contact the companies below.

NHM Worldwide Personal Imports
www.nhmworldwide.co.uk

Wellsprings
Eros House
Grand Rue, St. Martins
Guernsey
GY4 6LQ
Phone: +44 (0) 1481 233 370
Website: *www.wellsprings-health.com*
Email: *orders@wellsprings-health.com*

Wellsprings is based in the UK and it delivers progesterone globally. Make sure that you consult your health care practitioner before using any progesterone product obtained via import.

Finding a Doctor in the UK

For more information on progesterone in the UK or if you need help finding a doctor who prescribes progesterone (when appropriate), contact the organization below:

The Natural Progesterone Information Service
NPIS
P.O. Box 24
Buxton
SK17 9FB
Phone: 07000 784849
Website: *www.npis.info*
Email: *news@npis.info*
German Language: 0049- (0) 30-6939334
French Language: 01534 617587

References

Abramson, J. (2008). *Overdosed America: The Broken Promise of American Medicine.* New York: Harper Perennial.

Acs, P., Kipp, M., Norkute, A., Johann, S., Clarner, T., Braun, A., et al. (2009). 17beta-estradiol and progesterone prevent cuprizone provoked demyelination of corpus callosum in male mice. *Glia.* 57(8): 807-14.

Afifi, A., & Bergman, R. (2005). *Functional Neuroanatomy: Text and Atlas* (2nd ed.). Columbus, OH: McGraw-Hill Medical.

Barbaccia, M. L. (2004). Neurosteroidogenesis: relevance to neurosteroid actions in brain and modulaton by psychotropic drugs. *Critical Reviews in Neurobiology.* 16(1-2): 67-74.

Barbaccia, M. L., Serra, M., Purdy, R. H., & Biggio, G. (2001). Stress and neuroactive steroids. *International Review of Neurobiology.* 46: 243-72.

Baulieu, E. E. (1998). Neurosteroids: a novel function of the brain. *Psychoneuroendocrinology.* 23(8): 963-87.

Baulieu, E. E., & Robel, P. (1990). Neurosteroids: a new brain function? *The Journal of Steroid Biochemistry and Molecular Biology.* 37(3): 395-403.

Baulieu, E. E., Robel, P., & Schumacher, M. (2001). Neurosteroids: beginning of the story. *International Review of Neurobiology.* 46: 1-32.

Baulieu, E. E., & Schumacher, M. (2000). Progesterone as a neuroactive neurosteroid, with special reference to the effect of progesterone on myelination. *Steroids.* 65(10-11): 605-12.

Bernardi, F., Pluchino, N., Pieri, M., Begliuomini, S., Lenzi, E., Puccetti, S., et al. (2006). Progesterone and medroxyprogesterone acetate effects on central and peripheral allopregnanolone and beta-endorphin levels. *Neuroendocrinology.* 83(5-6): 348-59.

Bitran, D., Shiekh, M., & McLeod, M. (1995). Anxiolytic effect of progesterone is mediated by the neurosteroid allopregnanolone at brain GABAA receptors. *Journal of Neuroendocrinology.* 7(3): 171-7.

Calogero, A. E., Palumbo, M. A., Bosboom, A. M., Burrello, N., Ferrara, E., Palumbo, G., et al. (1998). The neuroactive steroid allopregnanolone suppresses hypothalamic gonadotropin-releasing hormone release through a mechanism mediated by the gamma-aminobutyric acidA receptor. *Journal of Endocrinology.* 158(1): 121-5.

Carre, J. L., Abalain, J. H., Sarlieve, L. L., & Floch, H. H. (2001). Ontogeny of steroid metabolizing enzymes in rat oligodendrocytes. *The Journal of Steroid Biochemistry and Molecular Biology.* 78(1): 89-95.

Carter, C. J. (2007). Multiple genes and factors associated with bipolar disorder converge on growth factor and stress activated kinase pathways controlling translation initiation: implications for oligodendrocyte viability. *Neurochemistry International.* 50(3): 461–490.

Celotti, F., Melcangi, R. C., & Martini, L. (1992). The 5 alpha-reductase in the brain: molecular aspects and relation to brain function. *Frontiers in Neuroendocrinology.* 13(2): 163-215.

Chan, J. R., Phillips, L. J. 2nd, & Glaser, M. (1998). Glucocorticoids and progestins signal the initiation and enhance the rate of myelin formation. *Proceedings of the National Academy of Sciences of the United States of America.* 95(18): 10459-64.

Charalampopoulos, I., Remboutsika, E., Margioris, A. N., & Gravanis, A. (2008). Neurosteroids as modulators of neurogenesis and neuronal survival. *Trends in Endocrinology & Metabolism.* 19(8): 300-7.

Chouinard, G., Steinberg, S., & Steiner, W. (1987, June). Estrogen-progesterone combination: another mood stabilizer? [Letter to the editor]. *The American Journal of Psychiatry.* 144(6): 826.

Ciriza, I., Carrero, P., Frye, C. A., & Garcia-Segura, L. M. (2006). Reduced metabolites mediate neuroprotective effects of progesterone in the adult rat hippocampus. The synthetic progestin medroxyprogesterone acetate (Provera) is not neuroprotective. *Journal of Neurobiology.* 66(9): 916-28.

Cotter, D., Mackay, D., Landau, S., Kerwin, R., & Everall, I. (2001). Reduced glial cell density and neuronal size in the anterior cingulate cortex in major depressive disorder. *Archives of General Psychiatry.* 58(6): 545-53.

Cotter, D. R., Pariante, C. M., & Everall, I. P. (2001). Glial cell abnormalities in major psychiatric disorders: the evidence and implications. *Brain Research Bulletin.* 55(5): 585-95.

Davis, K. L., Stewart, D. G., Friedman, J. I., Buchsbaum, M., Harvey, P. D., Hof, P. R., et al. (2003). White matter changes in schizophrenia: evidence for myelin-related dysfunction. *Archives of General Psychiatry.* 60(5): 443-56.

De Almeida, R. M., Ferrari, P. F., Parmigiani, S., & Miczek, K. A. (2005). Escalated aggressive behavior: dopamine, serotonin and GABA. *European Journal of Pharmacology*. 526(1-3): 51-64.

De Nicola, A. F., Labombarda, F., Gonzalez, S. L., Gonzalez Deniselle, M. C., Guennoun, R., & Schumacher, M. (2003). Steroid effects on glial cells: detrimental or protective for spinal cord function? *Annals of the New York Academy of Sciences*. 1007: 317-28.

Devinsky, O., & D'Esposito, M. (2004). *Neurology of Cognitve and Behavioral Disorders*. New York: Oxford University Press USA.

Dwork, A. J., Mancevski, B., & Rosoklija, G. (2007). White matter and cognitive function in schizophrenia. *International Journal of Neuropsychopharmacology*. 10(4): 513-36.

Engel, S. R., & Grant, K. A. (2001). Neurosteroids and behavior. *International Review of Neurobiology*. 46: 321-48.

Eser, D., Romeo, E., Baghai, T. C., di Michele, F., Schüle, C., Pasini, A., et al. (2006). Neuroactive steroids as modulators of depression and anxiety. *Neuroscience*. 138(3): 1041-8.

Eser, D., Romeo, E., Baghai, T. C., Schüle, C., Nothdurfter, C., & Rupprecht, R. (2008). Neuroactive steroids as endogenous modulators of anxiety. *Current Pharmaceutical Design*. 14(33): 3525-33.

Eser, D., Schüle, C., Baghai, T. C., Romeo, E., Uzunov, D. P., & Rupprecht, R. (2006). Neuroactive steroids and affective disorders. *Pharmacology, Biochemistry, and Behavior*. 84(4): 656-66.

Eva, C., Oberto, A., Mele, P., Serra, M., & Biggio, G. (2006). Role of brain neuroactive steroids in the functional interplay between the GABA(A) and the NPY-Y1 receptor mediated signals in the amygdala. *Pharmacology, Biochemistry, and Behavior.* 84(4): 568-80.

Feng, Y. (2008). Convergence and divergence in the etiology of myelin impairment in psychiatric disorders and drug addiction. *Neurochemical Research.* 33(10): 1940-9.

Flynn, S. W., Lang, D. J., Mackay, A. L., Goghari, V., Vavasour, I. M., Whittall, K. P., et al. (2003). Abnormalities of myelination in schizophrenia detected in vivo with MRI, and post-mortem with analysis of oligodendrocyte proteins. *Molecular Psychiatry.* 8(9): 811-20.

Gago, N., Akwa, Y., Sananès, N., Guennoun, R., Baulieu, E. E., El-Etr, M., et al. (2001). Progesterone and the oligodendroglial lineage: stage-dependent biosynthesis and metabolism. *Glia.* 36(3): 295-308.

Gallagher, J. P., Orozco-Cabal, L. F., Liu, J., & Shinnick-Gallagher, P. (2008). Synaptic physiology of central CRH system. *European Journal of Pharmacology.* 583(2-3): 215-25.

Gibbs, T. T., Russek, S. J., & Farb, D. H. (2006). Sulfated steroids as endogenous neuromodulators. *Pharmacology, Biochemistry, and Behavior.* 84(4): 555-6.7.

Girdler, S. S., & Klatzkin, R. (2007). Neurosteroids in the context of stress: implications for depressive disorders. *Pharmacology & Therapeutics.* 116(1): 125-39

Gogtay, N., Lu, A., Leow, A. D., Klunder, A. D, Chavez, A., Greenstein, D., et al. (2008). Three-dimensional brain growth abnormalities in childhood-onset schizophrenia visualized by using tensor-based morphometry. *Proceedings of the National Academy of Sciences of the United States of America.*
105(41): 15979-84.

Goldstein, J. M. (2006). Sex, hormones and affective arousal circuitry dysfunction in schizophrenia. *Hormones and Behavior.*
50(4): 612-22.

Haroutunian, V., & Davis, K. L. (2007). Introduction to the special section: myelin and oligodendrocyte abnormalities in schizophrenia. *The International Journal of Neuropsychopharmacology.*
10(4): 499-502.

Iversen, P. O., Stokland, A., Rolstad B., & Benestad, H. B. (1994). Adrenaline-induced leucocytosis: recruitment of blood cells from rat spleen, bone marrow and lymphatics. *European Journal of Applied Physiology and Occupational Physiology.*
68(3): 219-27.

Jefferies, W. M. (2004). *Safe Uses of Cortisol* (3rd ed.). Springfield, IL: Charles C. Thomas Publisher.

Katsel, P., Davis, K., & Haroutunian, V. (2005). Variations in myelin and oligodendrocyte-related gene expression across multiple brain regions in schizophrenia: a gene ontology study. *Schizophrenia Research.*
79(2-3): 157-173.

Kaur, P., Jodhka, P. K., Underwood, W. A., Bowles, C. A., de Fiebre, N. C., de Fiebre, C. M., et al. (2007). Progesterone increases brain-derived neuroptrophic factor expression and protects against glutamate toxicity in a mitogen-activated protein kinase- and phosphoinositide-3 kinase-dependent manner in cerebral cortical explants. *Journal of Neuroscience Research.*
85(11): 2441-9.

Koulen, P., Madry, C., Duncan, R. S., Hwang, J. Y., Nixon, E., McClung, N., et al. (2008). Progesterone potentiates IP (3)-mediated calcium signaling through Akt/PKB. *Cellular Physiology and Biochemistry.* 21(1-3): 161-72.

Lammers, C. H., Garcia-Borreguero, D., Schmider, J., Gotthardt, U., Dettling, M., Holsboer, F., et al. (1995). Combined dexamethasone/corticotropin-releasing hormone test in patients with schizophrenia and in normal controls: II. *Biological Psychiatry.* 38(12): 803-7.

Lee, J. R. (1999). *Natural Progesterone: The Multiple Roles of a Remarkable Hormone* (2nd ed.). Charlbury, the UK: Jon Carpenter Publishing.

Lee, J. R. (2003). *Hormone Balance for Men: What Your Doctor May Not Tell You About Prostate Health and Natural Hormone Supplementation.* Phoenix, AZ: Hormones Etc.

Lee, J. R., Hanley, J., & Hopkins, V. (1999). *What Your Doctor May Not Tell You About Premenopause: Balance Your Hormones and Your Life from Thirty to Fifty.* New York: Warner Books.

Lee, J. R., & Hopkins, V. (1996). *What Your Doctor May Not Tell You About Menopause: The Breakthrough Book on Natural Hormone Balance.* New York: Grand Central Publishing.

Lee, J. R., & Hopkins, V. (2006). *Dr. John Lee's Hormone Balance Made Simple: The Essential How-to-Guide to Symptoms, Dosage, Timing, and More.* New York: Wellness Central.

Liu, J., Yu, B., Neugebauer, V., Grigoriadis, D. E., Rivier, J., Vale, W. W., et al. (2004). Corticotropin-releasing factor and Urocortin I modulate excitatory glutamatergic synaptic transmission. *The Journal of Neuroscience.* 24(16): 4020-9.

MacKenzie, E. M., Odontiadis, J., Le Mellédo, J. M., Prior, T. I., & Baker, G. B. (2007). The relevance of neuroactive steroids in schizophrenia, depression, and anxiety disorders. *Cellular and Molecular Neurobiology.* 27(5): 541-74.

Martin, J. (2008). *Neuroanatomy: Text and Atlas* (3rd ed.). Columbus, OH: McGraw-Hill Medical.

Marx, C. E., Stevens, R. D., Shampine, L. J., Uzaunova, V., Trost, W. T., Butterfield, M. I., et al. (2006). Neuroactive steroids are altered in schizophrenia and bipolar disorder: relevance to pathophysiology and therapeutics. *Neuropsychopharmacology.* 31(6): 1249-63.

Maurice, T., Urani, A., Phan, V. L., & Romieu, P. (2001). The interaction between neuroactive steroids and the sigma 1 receptor function: behavioral consequences and therapeutic options. *Brain Research Reviews.* 37(1): 116-32.

Melcangi, R. C., Magnaghi, V., Galbiati, M., & Martini, L. (2001). Formation and effects of neuroactive steroids in the central and peripheral nervous system. *The International Review of Neurobiology.* 46: 145-76.

Mellon, S. H. (2007). Neurosteroid regulation of central nervous system development. *Pharmacology & Therapeutics.* 16(1): 107-24.

Miczek, K. A., Fish, E. W., & De Bold, J. F. (2003). Neurosteroids, GABAA receptors, and escalated aggressive behavior. *Hormones and Behavior.* 44(3): 242-57.

Ongür, D., Drevets, W. C., & Price, J. L. (1998). Glial reduction in the subgenual prefrontal cortex in mood disorders. *Proceedings of the National Academy of Sciences of the United States of America.* 95(22): 13290-5.

Orozco-Cabal, L., Pollandt, S., Liu, J., Shinnick-Gallagher, P., & Gallagher, J. P. (2006). Regulation of synaptic transmission by CRF receptors. *Reviews in the Neurosciences.* 17(3): 279-307.

Paul, S. M., & Purdy, R. H. (1992). Neuroactive steroids. *The Journal of the Federation of American Societies for Experimental Biology.* 6(6): 2311-22.

Pisu, M. G., & Serra, M. (2004). Neurosteroids and neuroactive drugs in mental disorders. *Life Sciences.*
74(26): 3181-97.

Platt, M. E. (2007). *The Miracle of Bio-Identical Hormones* (2nd ed.). Rancho Mirage, CA: Clancy Lane Publishing.

Pluchino, N., Luisi, M., Lenzi, E., Centofanti, M., Begliuomini, S., & Freschi, L. (2006). Progesterone and progestins: effects on brain, allopregnanolone and beta-endorphin. *The Journal of Steroid Biochemistry and Molecular Biology.*
102(1-5): 205-13.

Rasgon, N. L., Altshuler, L. L., Fairbanks, L., Elman, S., Bitran, J., Labarca, R., et al. (2005). Reproductive function and risk for PCOS in women treated for bipolar disorder. *Bipolar Disorders.*
7(3): 246-59.

Reddy, D. S. (2002). The clinical potentials of endogenous neurosteroids. *Drugs of Today.*
38(7): 465-85.

Reddy, D. S. (2003). Pharmacology of endogenous neuroactive steroids. *Critical Reviews in Neurobiology.*
15(3-4): 197-234.

Reddy, D. S. (2006). Physiological role of adrenal deoxycorticosterone-derived neuroactive steroids in stress-sensitive conditions. *Neuroscience.*
138(3): 911-20.

Reddy, D. S., & Kulkarni. S. K. (1998). The role of GABA-A and mitochondrial diazepam-binding inhibitor receptors on the effects of neurosteroids on food intake in mice. *Psychopharmacology.*
137(4): 391-400.

Regenold, W. T., Phatak, P., Marano, C. M., Gearhart, L., Viens, C. H., & Hisley, K. C. (2007). Myelin staining of deep white matter in the dorsolateral prefrontal cortex in schizophrenia, bipolar disorder, and unipolar major depression. *Psychiatry Research.*
151(3): 179-88.

Rhodes, M. E., Harney, J. P., & Frye, C. A. (2004). Gonadal, adrenal, and neuroactive steroids' role in ictal activity. *Brain Research.*
1000(1-2): 8-18.

Rupprecht, R. (2003). Neuroactive steroids: mechanisms of action and neuropsychopharmacological properties. *Psychoneuroendocrinology.*
28(2): 139-68.

Rupprecht, R., di Michele, F., Hermann, B., Ströhle, A., Lancel, M., Romeo, E., et al. (2001). Neuroactive steroids: molecular mechanisms of action and implications for neuropsychopharmacology. *Brain Research Reviews.*
37(1-3): 59-67.

Rupprecht, R., & Holsboer, F. (1999). Neuropsychopharmacological properties of neuroactive steroids. *Steroids.*
64(1-2): 83-91.

Rupprecht, R., & Holsboer, F. (2001). Neuroactive steroids in neuropsychopharmacology. *International Review of Neurobiology.*
46: 461-77.

Rupprecht, R., Reul, J. M., Trapp, T., van Steensel, B., Wetzel, C., Damm, K., et al. (1993). Progesterone receptor-mediated effects of neuroactive steroids. *Neuron.*
11(3): 523-30.

Rushton, A. (2003). *Natural Progesterone: The Natural Way to Alleviate Symptoms of Menopause, PMS, and other Hormone-Related Problems.* London: Thorsons.

Schumacher, M., Akwa, Y., Guennoun, R., Robert, F., Labombarda, F., Desarnaud, F., et al. (2000). Steroid synthesis and metabolism in the nervous system: trophic and protective effects. *Journal of Neurocytology.*
29(5-6): 307-26.

Schumacher, M., Guennoun, R., Robert, F., Carelli, C., Gago, N., Ghoumari, A., et al. (2004). Local synthesis and dual actions of progesterone in the nervous system: neuroprotection and myelination. *Growth Hormone & IGF Research.*
14 Suppl A: S18-33.

Segal, D., Koschnick, J. R., Slegers, L. H., & Hof, P. R. (2007). Oligodendrocyte pathophysiology: a new view of schizophrenia. *The International Journal of Neuropsychopharmacology.*
10(4): 503-11.

Shealy, C. N. (1999). *Natural Progesterone Cream: Safe and Natural Hormone Replacement.* Columbus, OH: McGraw-Hill.

Shulman, Y., & Tibbo, P. G. (2005). Neuroactive steroids in schizophrenia. *The Canadian Journal of Psychiatry.*
50(11): 695- 702.

Simpkins, J. W., Yang, S. H., Wen, Y., & Singh, M. (2005). Estrogens, progestins, menopause and neurodegeneration: basic and clinical studies. *Cellular and Molecular Life Sciences.*
62(3): 271-80.

Singh, M. (2005). Mechanisms of progesterone-induced neuroprotection. *Annals of the New York Academy of Sciences.*
1052: 145-51.

Singh, M. (2006). Progesterone-induced neuroprotection. *Endocrine.*
29(2): 271-4.

Singh, M., Meyer, E. M., Millard, W. J., & Simpkins, J. W. (1994). Ovarian steroid deprivation results in a reversible learning impairment and compromised cholinergic function in female Sprague-Dawley rats. *Brain Research.*
644(2): 305-12.

Singh, M., Sumien, N., Kyser, C., & Simpkins, J. W. (2008). Estrogens and progesterone as neuroprotectants: what animal models teach us. *Frontiers in Bioscience.*
13: 1083-9

Smith, S. S. (2006). Withdrawal properties of a neuroactive steroid: implications for GABA(A) receptor gene regulation in the brain and anxiety behavior. *Steroids.*
67(6): 519-28.

Strous, R. D., Maayan, R., & Weizman, A. (2006). The relevance of neurosteroids to clinical psychiatry: from the laboratory to the bedside. *European Neuropsychopharmacology.*
16(3): 155-69.

Stuss, D. T., Winocur, G., & Robertson, I. H. (1999). *Cognitive Neurorehabiliation.* Cambridge, the UK: Cambridge University Press.

Tkachev, D., Mimmack, M. L., Huffaker, S. J., Ryan, M., & Bahn, S. (2007). Further evidence for altered myelin biosynthesis and glutamatergic dysfunction in schizophrenia. *The International Journal of Neuropsychopharmacology.*
10(4): 557-563.

Tkachev, D., Mimmack, M. L., Ryan, M. M., Wayland, M., Freeman, T., Jones, P. B., et al. (2003). Oligodendrocyte dysfunction in schizophrenia and bipolar disorder. *The Lancet.*
362(9386): 798-805.

Torres, J. M., & Ortega, E. (2003). DHEA, PREG and their sulphate derivatives on plasma and brain after CRH and ACTH administration. *Neurochemical Research.*
28(8): 1187-91.

Ugale, R. R., Hirani, K., Morelli, M., & Chopde, C. T. (2004). Role of neuroactive steroid allopregnanolone in antipsychotic-like action of olanzapine in rodents. *Neuropsychopharmacology.*
29(9): 1597-609.

Uranova, N. A., Vostrikov, V. M., Orlovskaya, D. D., & Rachmanova, V. I. (2004). Oligodendroglial density in the prefrontal cortex in schizophrenia and mood disorders: a study from the Stanley Neuropathology Consortium. *Schizophrenia Research.*
67(2-3): 269-75.

Uranova, N. A., Vostrikov, V. M., Vikhreva, O. V., Zimina, I. S., Kolomeets, N. S., & Orlovskaya, D. D. (2007). The role of oligodendrocyte pathology in schizophrenia. *International Journal of Neuropsychopharmacology.*
10(4): 537-45.

Uzunova, V., Sampson, L., & Uzunov, D. P. (2006). Relevance of endogenous 3alpha-reduced neurosteroids to depression and antidepressant action. *Psychopharmacology.*
186(3): 351-61.

Vallée, M., Mayo, W., Koob, G. F., & Le Moal, M. (2001). Neurosteroids in learning and memory processes. *International Review of Neurobiology.*
46: 273-320.

Viero, C., & Dayanithi, G. (2008). Neurosteroids are excitatory in supraoptic neurons but inhibitory in the peripheral nervous system: it is all about oxytocin and progesterone receptors. *Progress in Brain Research.*
170: 177-92.

Vostrikov, V., Orlovskaya, D., & Uranova, N. (2008). Deficit of pericapillary oligodendrocytes in the prefrontal cortex in schizophrenia. *The World Journal of Biological Psychiatry.*
9(1): 34-42.

Walker, E. F., Bonsall, R., & Walder, D. J. (2002). Plasma hormones and catecholamine metabolites in monozygotic twins discordant for psychosis. *Neuropsychiatry, Neuropsychology, and Behavioral Neurology.*
15(1): 10-7.

Wieck, A., Davies, R. A., Hirst, A. D., Brown, N., Papadopoulos, A., Marks, M. N., et al. (2003). Menstrual cycle effects on hypothalamic dopamine receptor function in women with a history of puerperal bipolar disorder. *Journal of Psychopharmacology.*
17(2): 204-9.

Williams, K. E., Marsh, W. K., & Rasgon, N. L. (2007). Mood disorders and fertility in women: a critical review of the literature and implications for future research. *Human Reproduction Update.*
13(6): 607-16.

Wilson, J. L. (2002). *Adrenal Fatigue: The 21st Century Stress Syndrome*. Petaluma, CA: Smart Publications.

Yim, I. S., Glynn, L. M., Dunkel-Schetter, C., Hobel, C. J., Chicz-DeMet, A., & Sandman, C. A. (2009). Risk of postpartum depressive symptoms with elevated corticotropin-releasing hormone in human pregnancy. *Archives of General Psychiatry.* 66(2): 162-9.

Zinder, O., & Dar, D. E. (1999). Neuroactive steroids: their mechanism of action and their function in the stress response. *Acta Physiologica Scandinavica.* 167(3): 181-8.

Index

adrenal glands	20, 22
adrenaline	21
allergies	27
aldosterone	20-21
amenorrhea	44
antidepressants	62
antipsychotics	62
anxiety disorders	19, 21
attention deficit disorder	64-65
auditory hallucinations	19
autoimmune disease	21, 64
bioidentical progesterone	24, 28-31, 36-37, 63
bipolar disorder	11, 13, 19, 64, 68
birth control pills	43, 58
blood pressure	21
blood sugar	21, 46
brain stem	18-19
calendar	42, 44
cancer	66
candida	63

cerebellum	17-18
children	65
compounding pharmacy	35, 58
concentration	13, 21
cortisol	20-21
delusions	14
depression	13-14
digestive disorder	63
DNA (deoxyribonucleic acid)	64
epinephrine	*see adrenaline*
estradiol	26
estrogen	22, 26, 48-49, 52, 54
family doctor	11, 58
fatigue	15, 21, 63
Food and Drug Administration (FDA)	44, 67
frontal lobe	18-19
gynecologist	58
hallucinations	14, 19
hormone replacement therapy (HRT)	47-48, 58
hypogonadism	22

impulse control	13, 18
insulin	23, 65
internist	65
irregular cycles (menstrual)	46
juvenile diabetes	23, 65
liver	31
limbic system	18-19
loading dose	39, 42
lymph nodes	21, 65
mania	13-14, 21
medroxyprogesterone acetate	30
memory	15, 18
menopause	48-49
menstruation	38, 42
mood stabilizers	62
myelin (sheath)	68
neuron(s)	17, 68
occipital lope	18-19
oral progesterone	66
osteoporosis	27, 51
ovaries	22

parietal lobe	18-19
pharmaceutical companies	69
polycystic ovaries	27
pregnancy	43, 52, 67
premenstrual dysphoric disorder (PMDD)	46
premenstrual syndrome (PMS)	46
prescription	35-36, 50, 66, 69
progesterone	11, 19-22, 24-26, 28, 49, 52,-54, 62-64
progestins	28, 30, 66-67
Prometrium	66
Provera	*see medroxyprogesterone acetate*
psychiatric medications	55, 62, 69
psychiatry	62
racing thoughts	13
saliva test	25
schizophrenia	11, 14-15, 19, 64, 68
senators	69-70
sexual characteristics	52
synthetic progesterone	*see progestins*
temporal lobes	18-19
testosterone	50, 52

transdermal progesterone	**31, 33, 38**
type 1 diabetes	*see juvenile diabetes*
uterine lining	**50, 64**
visual hallucinations	**19**
xenoestrogens	**67**
yellow pages	**58**
ZRT Laboratory	**25, 59**

ABOUT THE AUTHOR

Doris King was born in Winter Haven, Florida and raised in Lake Alfred, Florida. She graduated from Auburndale High School and attended college at Florida A&M University in Tallahassee, Florida. After graduation, Doris taught school in metro Atlanta. Today she lives and works in Central Florida. Doris suffered from symptoms of bipolar disorder and schizophrenia for over 20 years. Today she is symptom-free because she takes progesterone.

TO CONTACT THE AUTHOR:
Email: *doris@dorisking.net*
Web: *www.dorisking.net*

ACKNOWLEDGEMENTS

Thank you to my wonderful editor, Aileen Cho—I could not have finished this book without you. To the estate of Dr. John Lee—my gratitude is yours for allowing me to reprint so much of his work.

To my parents, Laveral and Helen—thank you for your constant love and support. To my brother and sister, Laveral Jr. "Man" and Eva—thank you for always believing in me.

To my nieces and nephews—Kurt, Kaiya, Kassidy, Kenard, Karalyn, Malik, Mia, and Jayden—thank you for being so much fun and for making my life so bright.

I also thank a host of friends, family, and colleagues who continuously supported me throughout this book-writing journey. Thank you to my Aunt Queen King, Dr. Betty Freeman, Kardawn Floyd, Gail Cooper, Ursula Morrow, Nancy Bush, Anitra McKnight, Anthony Gilpin, Tracy Thompson, Charman Green, and Robyn Donaldson. Your constant support has been invaluable to me.

And a special thank you to Rachel Bergman, who implemented the final changes to my text and helped me down the home stretch—I appreciate all your help and assistance in completing this project.

CPSIA information can be obtained at www.ICGtesting.com
Printed in the USA
LVOW06s1245150814

399230LV00001B/43/P

9 780982 485309